A Moment Just For Me

Finding the calm amidst the chaos

Dementia Doulas Australia
By Wendy Hall

The information and conversations in this book have been set down to the best of the author's ability. This book does not contain medical advice and is not a substitute for professional support.

Copyright © 2025 by Dementia Doulas International

All rights reserved. No part of this book may be reproduced or used in any manner without written permission of the copyright owner except for the use of quotations in a book review. For more information, address: hello@dementiadoulas.org.au

First paperback edition October 2025

Book cover design by Daria DiCieli

Author: Wendy Hall

ISBN: 978-0-6451185-4-4 (paperback)

www.dementiadoulas.org.au

CHAPTERS

WHAT THE WORLD CANNOT SEE	11
MORE THAN A LABEL	21
HONOURING MY STORY	31
THE ME I'M BECOMING	41
THE WARMTH OF A MEMORY	51
NAMING MY NEEDS	61
GROWING THROUGH CHANGE	71
PERMISSION TO FEEL IT ALL	81
WHAT REST LOOKS LIKE FOR ME	91
TENDING TO MY FRAYED EDGES	101
LITTLE JOYS, BIG IMPACT	111
BOUNDARIES ARE KINDNESS	121
TINY SPARKS OF HOPE	131
MOMENTS I WANT TO KEEP	141
WHAT I STILL DREAM ABOUT	151
LIFE BEYOND THE ROLE	161

Dear You,

This journal is for the part of you that often gets tucked away beneath the weight of responsibility, routine, and love. It's for the part that existed before the caring role and will remain long after it shifts or fades. You are more than a 'carer'. You are someone with dreams, desires, memories, and a future that is still unfolding.

In the quiet moments between medications and meals, between appointments and phone calls, I invite you to reconnect with yourself. To honour the wife, husband, partner, mother, father, daughter, son, friend, who is you. You are so much more than the label of 'carer'. You matter not just for what you do, but for who you are.

This journal is designed to be a safe place to pause, breathe, reflect and remember. It's a gentle reminder that your wellbeing is not a luxury, it's a lifeline. And that rediscovering yourself is not an act of selfishness, but an act of survival, healing, and hope.

There will come a time, perhaps already here, perhaps still distant, when the intensity of your caring role softens or ends. When that time comes, may you not feel lost. May you feel prepared and may you feel held by all the parts of yourself you nurtured along the way.

So take the space this journal offers and make it yours. Write in it honestly, cry into its pages and dream between the lines. Let this be a map back to you!

With warmth, respect and deep admiration,

Wendy Hall

Wendy Hall
Dementia Doulas Australia

Your Emotional & Mental Health

Taking on a care role, regardless of whether it happens suddenly or over time, can often come with a range of feelings and emotions. Many say that once a diagnosis of a condition has been identified, feelings of love and protection for the person increased. At the same time, some feel a sense of helplessness because they can't control or improve the situation.

Common feelings at various stages of the journey include:
• fear • confusion • guilt • blame • uncertainty • insecurity

All of these feelings are common, and normal. There's no such thing as a wrong feeling and speaking to a counsellor, therapist or health professional may help you understand and work through your emotions, and develop coping skills.

Here are some things you can do to help:

Cry: it seems obvious, but crying helps get the emotions out, it triggers the body to release chemicals that will help you feel better.

Keep a journal: a journal or diary is a private space just for you, express anything you want, knowing no one but you will read it.

Talk: if you have a trusted friend or family member, ask them if they can be a person you come to with big feelings.

Do things that make you happy: finding even a tiny amount of time to do little things for yourself can make a big difference.

Tread carefully before making decisions: if you're overtired or distressed, it can strongly affect your decision-making skills.

Be kind to yourself: it's okay to let feelings come and go without judging yourself.

Adapted from: The beyondblue Guide for Carers – Supporting and caring for a person with depression, anxiety and/or a related disorder

Chapter 1
WHAT THE WORLD CANNOT SEE

When you allow yourself a fresh start, even in tiny ways, you remind yourself that life still holds possibility. New beginnings create hope and help you feel less stuck.

Every day is a new beginning, though it rarely feels that way when life is full of routines and responsibilities. This chapter is an invitation to see small moments as fresh starts, tiny chances to choose kindness for yourself. You don't need to overhaul your world; you only need to allow yourself one new beginning that feels gentle and possible.

This book is a soft-landing, a space just for you, beyond tasks, to-do lists, and the constant 'what's next?' You're more than the role you've been asked to play. You're someone who feels deeply, remembers quietly, and carries more than most people ever see. Let these pages be a companion, a witness, and a gentle reminder that you matter not just for what you do, but for who you are.

Small Self-Care Suggestion:

Look at an old photo or listen to music from a time you felt most 'you.'

MY GENTLE GOAL FOR THIS CHAPTER

If the thought of big goals feels heavy, choose one thing you'd like to try sometime soon. It might be opening a window each morning, or writing one word to describe how you want to feel in the coming weeks.

My gentle goal is:

How I'll know I honoured it:

I give myself permission to choose one simple thing that feels possible for me right now. It doesn't need to be big or perfect. Small is enough.

Moment for Reflection:

Who was I before this journey began?

What parts of me are still here, waiting to be seen?

GRATITUDE JOURNAL

The best part of the day was:
_____

3 good things that happened today:

- _____
- _____
- _____

People I'm grateful for:

- _____
- _____
- _____

3 things I'm grateful for today:

- _____
- _____
- _____

Tomorrow, I'm looking forward to:
_____
_____
_____

Moment for Reflection:

A letter to myself – If my mind and body could write me a letter, what would it thank me for?

What would it ask me for more of?

SELF-CARE CHECKLIST

Self-care isn't just the act of ticking a box, it's a commitment to oneself. How did you look after yourself this week?

- [ ] Take a long bath
- [ ] Read for pleasure
- [ ] Go for a long walk
- [ ] Mindful meditation
- [ ] Journal thoughts
- [ ] Try gentle yoga
- [ ] Cook a meal
- [ ] Visit a museum/gallery
- [ ] Gardening
- [ ] Paint or draw
- [ ] Engage in a hobby
- [ ] Listen to favorite music
- [ ] Spend time with a friend
- [ ] Watch a movie
- [ ] Pamper yourself
- [ ] Take a short nap
- [ ] Go for a swim
- [ ] Practice gratitude
- [ ] Attend a workshop
- [ ] Explore a new place

Moment for Reflection:

Every sunrise is a chance to begin again. I will find a beginning that feels kind and possible for me.

Moment for Reflection:

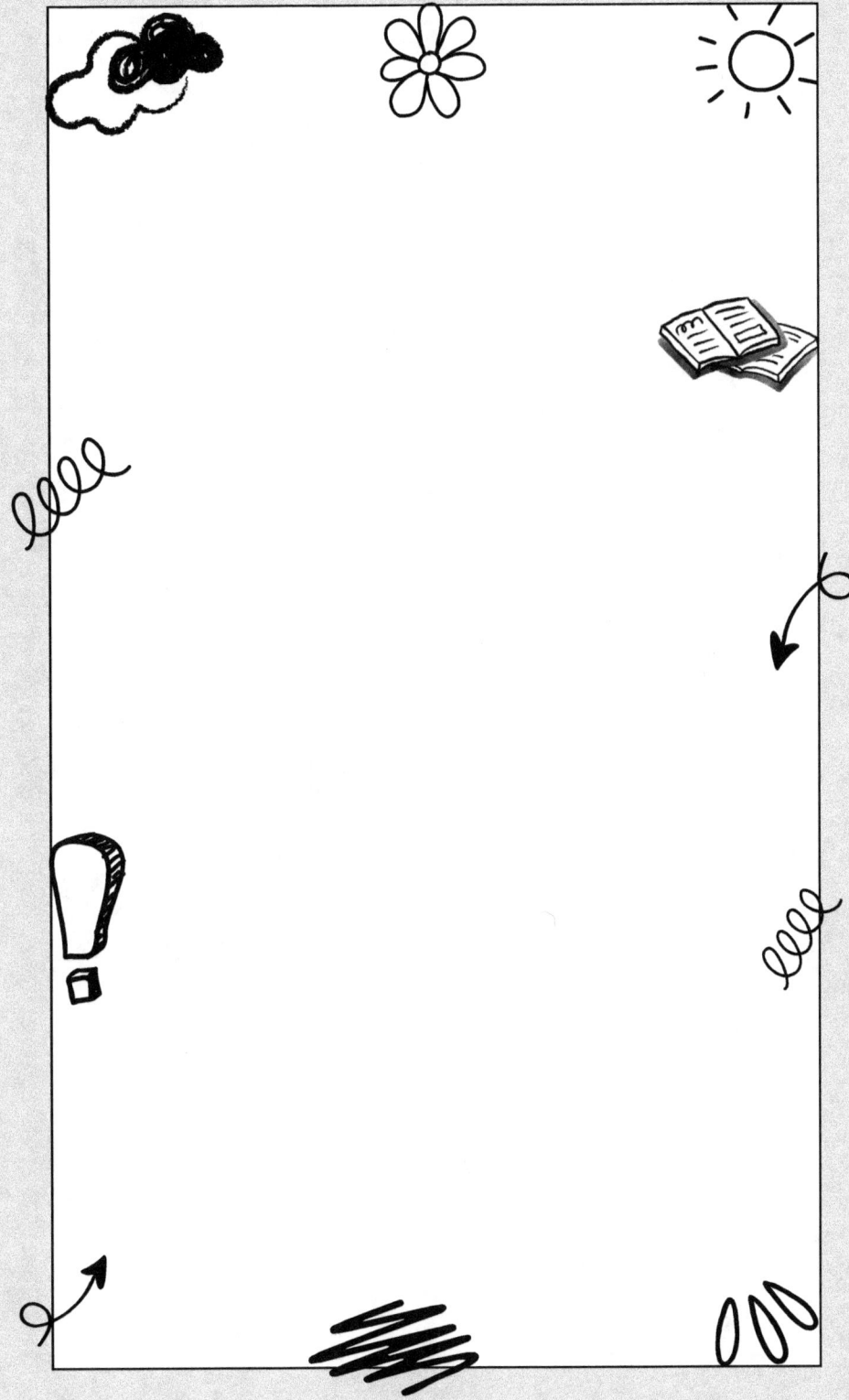

Chapter 2
MORE THAN A LABEL

I am not just one thing, I am layers, seasons and stories.

Your worth isn't measured purely by tasks or titles you may feel have been assigned to you. You existed long before this role, and the person you are should not be lost within the caring journey.

Caring can sometimes feel like holding your breath, waiting for the next call, the next task, the next need. This chapter is about reclaiming your breath, even if only for a few minutes. Breathing space doesn't have to be long; it can be a pause, a cup of tea in silence, or a slow exhale, that reminds you you're here, too.

In the care of others, it's easy to lose sight of yourself, but know you're not invisible here. This is time to honour the parts of you that have waited patiently in the background: the creative, the dreamer, the adventurer, the one who danced in kitchens and laughed until you cried. Those parts of you are still here to explore again, slowly, kindly, and without pressure.

Small Self-Care Suggestion:
Place one hand over your heart and the other on your stomach.
- Inhale slowly through your nose for a count of four, and feel your stomach rise. Hold for a count of four.
- Exhale softly through your mouth for a count of six and let your shoulders drop. Repeat this three times.

MY GENTLE GOAL FOR THIS CHAPTER

Taking a few minutes to pause and breathe, helps to reduce stress and bring a sense of clarity. Focus on breathing is like medicine for your mind and body and gives you time to reset. Taking moments to breathe deeply lowers stress, steadies your mind, and restores calm.

One small pause I will try is ...

How I'll know I honoured it:

I give myself permission to choose one simple thing that feels possible for me right now. It doesn't need to be big or perfect. Small is enough.

Moment for Reflection:

What roles do I play and what parts of me get lost in the label of 'carer'?

What brings me energy or joy that has nothing to do with caring?

GRATITUDE JOURNAL

The best part of the day was:
_____

3 good things that happened today:

- _____
- _____
- _____

People I'm grateful for:

- _____
- _____
- _____

3 things I'm grateful for today:

- _____
- _____
- _____

Tomorrow, I'm looking forward to:
_____
_____
_____

Moment for Reflection:

What would it look like to give myself two minutes of breathing space today?

What prompt can I use to remind me to pause for a moment?

SELF-CARE CHECKLIST

Self-care isn't just the act of ticking a box, it's a commitment to oneself. How did you look after yourself this week?

- [ ] Take a long bath
- [ ] Read for pleasure
- [ ] Go for a long walk
- [ ] Mindful meditation
- [ ] Journal thoughts
- [ ] Try gentle yoga
- [ ] Cook a meal
- [ ] Visit a museum/gallery
- [ ] Gardening
- [ ] Paint or draw
- [ ] Engage in a hobby
- [ ] Listen to favorite music
- [ ] Spend time with a friend
- [ ] Watch a movie
- [ ] Pamper yourself
- [ ] Take a short nap
- [ ] Go for a swim
- [ ] Practice gratitude
- [ ] Attend a workshop
- [ ] Explore a new place

Moment for Reflection:

Even the smallest pause is enough. May your breath remind you that you, too, deserve space to simply be.

Moment for Reflection:

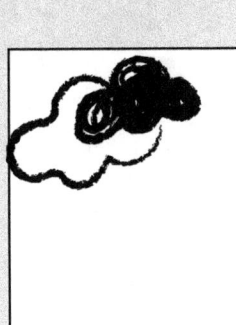

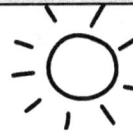

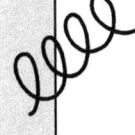
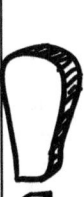
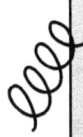
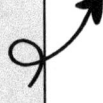
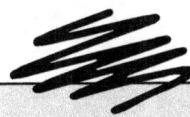
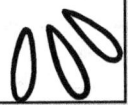

Give it a try:

Write your name in the middle of this page and surround it with words that describe your other identities (artist, writer, gardener, friend, etc.)

Chapter 3
HONOURING MY STORY

You don't need to be 'fine' to be worthy of honour.

Life is made up of seasons, some busy, some slow, some heavy, some light. When you are in a care role, it can be easy to feel stuck in one season without choice. This chapter encourages you to notice the season you're in now, and to honour it without judgment. Seasons shift and so will this one. Every season brings its own rhythm, some are bright with energy, others are slow and cooler.

There's no need to rush, no need to make any decisions or changes before you're ready. Allow yourself permission to simply 'be', to name the weight you carry, and to sit with your truth. It's a time to listen for your own voice beneath the noise, to acknowledge whatever you're feeling and know it's valid.

By honouring the season you're in, you release the fight against yourself. You are enabled to release guilt, lean into acceptance, and find gentleness in each moment. Accepting 'this is where I am', reduces unnecessary pressure and creates space for self-kindness.

Small Self-Care Suggestion:
Choose one meal this week that is just for you.
- Prepare it with intention then sit, breathe, and eat slowly
- Notice how your body feels when it is cared for

MY GENTLE GOAL FOR THIS CHAPTER

Simply sitting down with a meal instead of eating on the run, or adding one fresh piece of fruit to your day, is a way to honour yourself and give you some time.

One choice I will make just for myself is …

How I'll know I honoured it:

I give myself permission to choose one simple thing that feels possible for me right now. It doesn't need to be big or perfect. Small is enough.

Moment for Reflection:

What events in my life have shaped me, strengthened me, softened me?

What chapters of my story deserve to be honoured and not hidden?

GRATITUDE JOURNAL

The best part of the day was:
_____

3 good things that happened today:

- _____
- _____
- _____

People I'm grateful for:

- _____
- _____
- _____

3 things I'm grateful for today:

- _____
- _____
- _____

Tomorrow, I'm looking forward to:
_____
_____
_____

Moment for Reflection:

How does this season of caring feel in my body?

What food, movement, or routine helps me stay steady in this stage?

SELF-CARE CHECKLIST

Self-care isn't just the act of ticking a box, it's a commitment to oneself. How did you look after yourself this week?

- [ ] Take a long bath
- [ ] Engage in a hobby
- [ ] Read for pleasure
- [ ] Listen to favorite music
- [ ] Go for a long walk
- [ ] Spend time with a friend
- [ ] Mindful meditation
- [ ] Watch a movie
- [ ] Journal thoughts
- [ ] Pamper yourself
- [ ] Try gentle yoga
- [ ] Take a short nap
- [ ] Cook a meal
- [ ] Go for a swim
- [ ] Visit a museum/gallery
- [ ] Practice gratitude
- [ ] Gardening
- [ ] Attend a workshop
- [ ] Paint or draw
- [ ] Explore a new place

Moment for Reflection:

Seasons shift in their own time. May you find peace in the one you are in, trusting that change will come gently when it's ready.

Moment for Reflection:

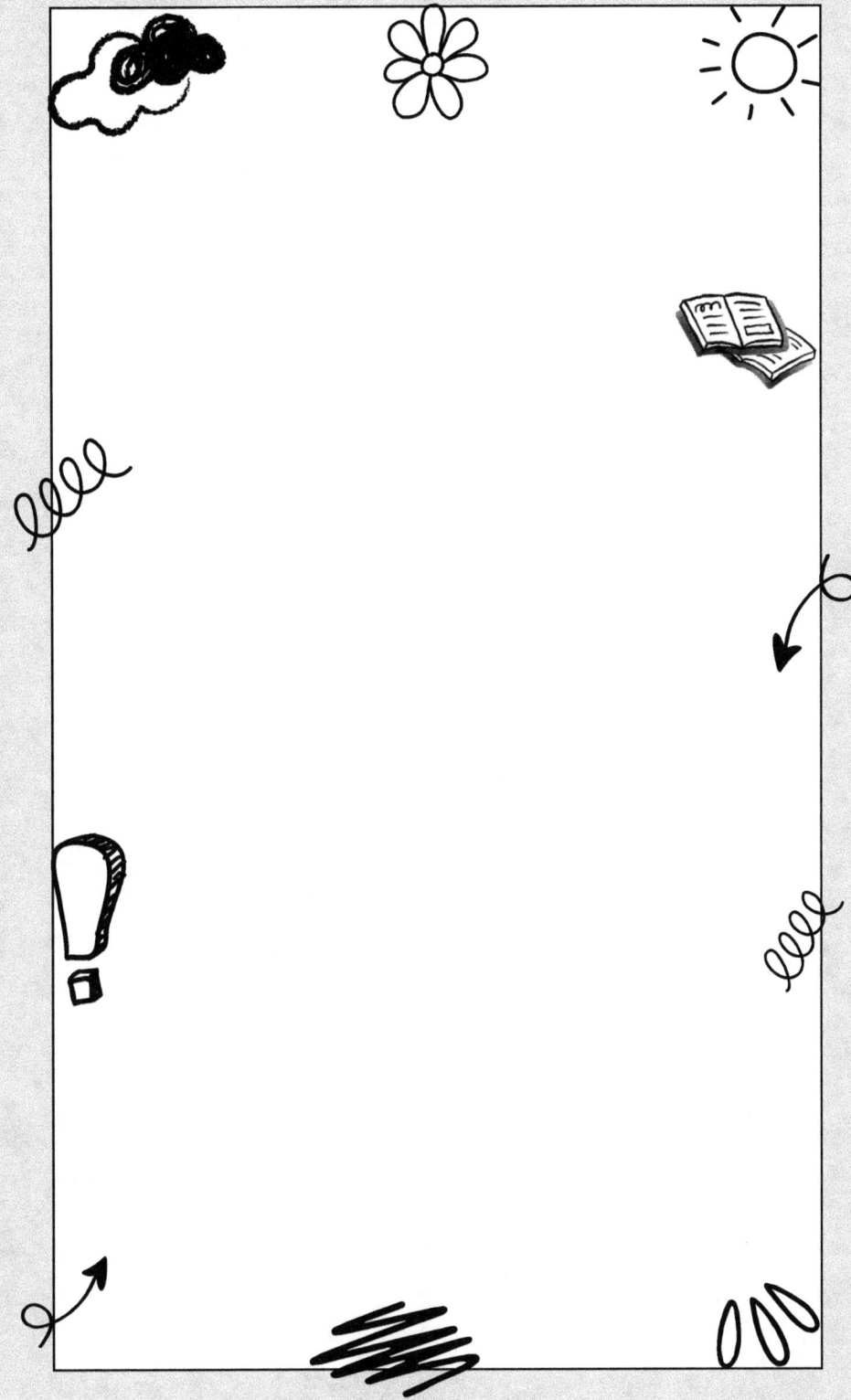

Chapter 4
THE ME I'M BECOMING

You're still becoming who you're meant to be, even now, especially now.

When life feels like it's swirling around you, it helps to have something to hold onto. Each week offers you a small anchor, a theme to explore, a practice to try, a prompt to reflect on. Let it meet you wherever you are, there's no pressure to 'get it right.' These aren't tasks. They're invitations to slow down, to notice, to breathe, to come home to yourself, one moment at a time.

Your body holds the weight of caring, often without being asked. Movement doesn't need to mean exercise. It can mean stretching your arms, taking a gentle walk, or swaying to music in your kitchen. This chapter invites you to move with kindness, not to achieve, but to release.

Gentle movement restores energy, eases tension and helps your body carry less of the weight of caring, it can boost mood and strengthen resilience. It can make your body feel lighter, and allow your energy to grow, even with the smallest stretches. It's a perfect way of giving back to yourself.

Small Self-Care Suggestion:

Write a letter to yourself from a place of deep compassion.

MY GENTLE GOAL FOR THIS CHAPTER

More movement during the day is a way to nurture your body and clear your mind. It might be; a slow stretch while the kettle boils, a walk to the letterbox or in the garden, or dancing to your favourite song for just two minutes.

One gentle movement I will gift myself is ...

How I'll know I honoured it:

I give myself permission to choose one simple thing that feels possible for me right now. It doesn't need to be big or perfect. Small is enough.

Moment for Reflection:

Who am I evolving into, and how do I feel about that?

In what ways have I grown or surprised myself lately?

GRATITUDE JOURNAL

The best part of the day was:
_____

3 good things that happened today:

- _____
- _____
- _____

People I'm grateful for:

- _____
- _____
- _____

3 things I'm grateful for today:

- _____
- _____
- _____

Tomorrow, I'm looking forward to:
_____
_____
_____

Moment for Reflection:

What's one small way I can move kindly today, rolling my shoulders, or walking to the letterbox and back?

What is one small, intentional act I can repeat this week to feel grounded, whether a walk, a meal, or a mindful pause?

SELF-CARE CHECKLIST

Self-care isn't just the act of ticking a box, it's a commitment to oneself. How did you look after yourself this week?

- ☐ Take a long bath
- ☐ Read for pleasure
- ☐ Go for a long walk
- ☐ Mindful meditation
- ☐ Journal thoughts
- ☐ Try gentle yoga
- ☐ Cook a meal
- ☐ Visit a museum/gallery
- ☐ Gardening
- ☐ Paint or draw
- ☐ Engage in a hobby
- ☐ Listen to favorite music
- ☐ Spend time with a friend
- ☐ Watch a movie
- ☐ Pamper yourself
- ☐ Take a short nap
- ☐ Go for a swim
- ☐ Practice gratitude
- ☐ Attend a workshop
- ☐ Explore a new place

Moment for Reflection:

Movement will keep life flowing through me softly and steadily.

Moment for Reflection:

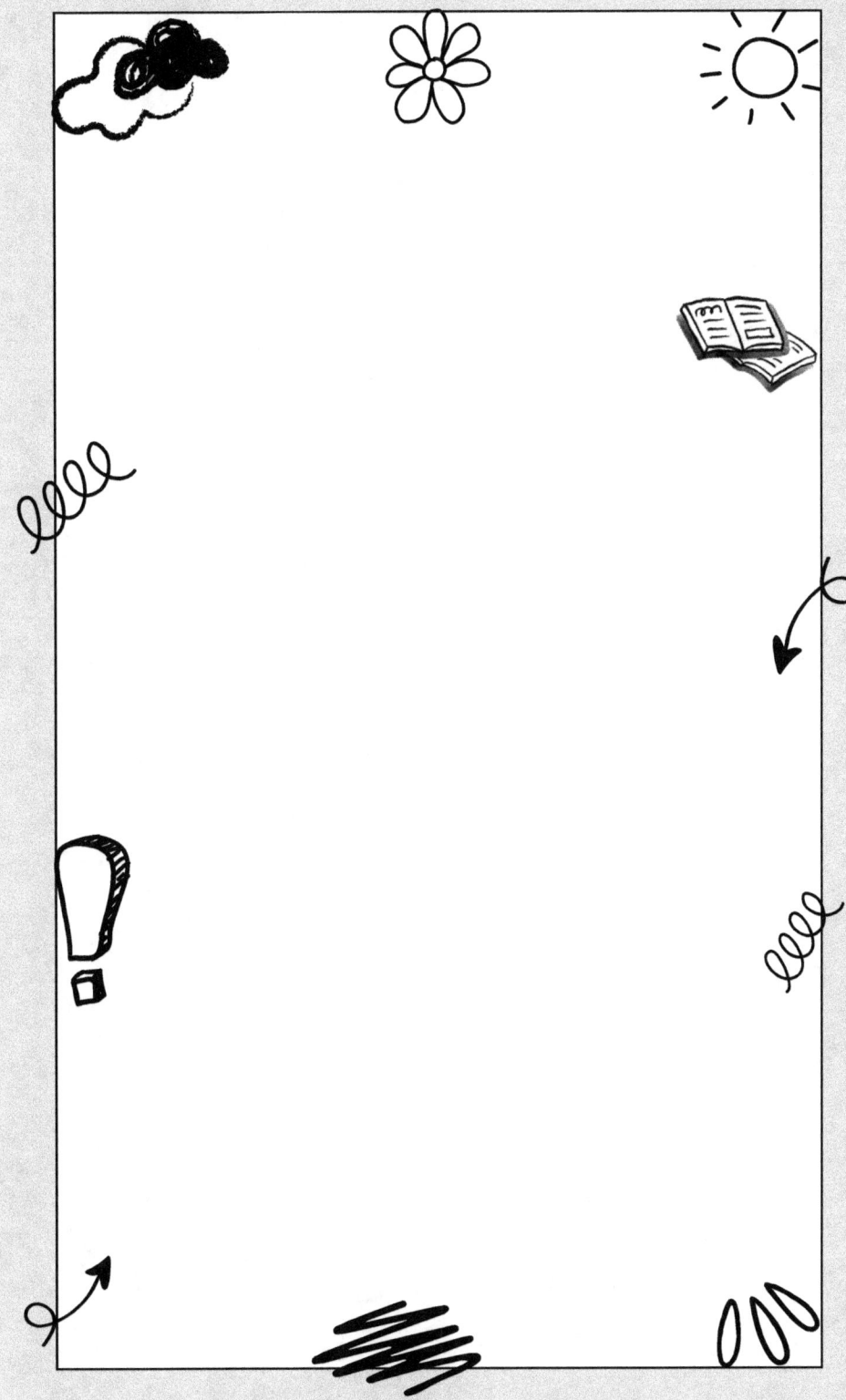

Chapter 5
THE WARMTH OF A MEMORY

Just because you carry it well doesn't mean it's not heavy.

Food is a memory all on its own. A simple scent, a warm bowl, a familiar flavour can bring us back to the people and places that shaped us. This chapter isn't about perfection or health plans, it's about comfort. The kind that lives in your favourite mug, or the steam from something cooked slowly with love. Here, we reconnect through the rituals, and the warmth of nourishing yourself.

Food can carry so many memories while bringing a warmth, and grounding. The kitchen can feel like another place of duty, but it can also become a source of comfort. This can come from the simple nourishment through tastes that remind you of safety, recipes that bring smiles, or quiet moments of preparing something just for you.

Nourishing food restores your strength and stabilises your mood. Cooking or enjoying comfort food reconnects you to memory and pleasure and not just to duty. Nourishing yourself through food improves energy, mood, and focus.

Small Self-Care Suggestion:

Bring something fresh into your kitchen this week, a sprig of parsley, a lemon, or even a flower in a glass.

MY GENTLE GOAL FOR THIS CHAPTER

Let your goal be one small act of grounding through food or plants.

One kitchen or garden ritual I will try is ...

How I'll know I honoured it:

I give myself permission to choose one simple thing that feels possible for me right now. It doesn't need to be big or perfect. Small is enough.

Moment for Reflection:

What am I holding that I haven't put into words?

What emotional weight am I carrying quietly right now?

GRATITUDE JOURNAL

The best part of the day was:
_____

3 good things that happened today:

- _____
- _____
- _____

People I'm grateful for:

- _____
- _____
- _____

3 things I'm grateful for today:

- _____
- _____
- _____

Tomorrow, I'm looking forward to:
_____
_____
_____

Moment for Reflection:

What meal makes me feel calm, strong, or joyful?

Could I prepare it in a way that also supports my health? (For eg. preparing a meal with others or shopping at a local market)

SELF-CARE CHECKLIST

Self-care isn't just the act of ticking a box, it's a commitment to oneself. How did you look after yourself this week?

- [ ] Take a long bath
- [ ] Read for pleasure
- [ ] Go for a long walk
- [ ] Mindful meditation
- [ ] Journal thoughts
- [ ] Try gentle yoga
- [ ] Cook a meal
- [ ] Visit a museum/gallery
- [ ] Gardening
- [ ] Paint or draw
- [ ] Engage in a hobby
- [ ] Listen to favorite music
- [ ] Spend time with a friend
- [ ] Watch a movie
- [ ] Pamper yourself
- [ ] Take a short nap
- [ ] Go for a swim
- [ ] Practice gratitude
- [ ] Attend a workshop
- [ ] Explore a new place

Moment for Reflection:

Food is more than fuel; it is comfort, memory, and connection. May you taste warmth and feel nourished in ways that go beyond the table.

Moment for Reflection:

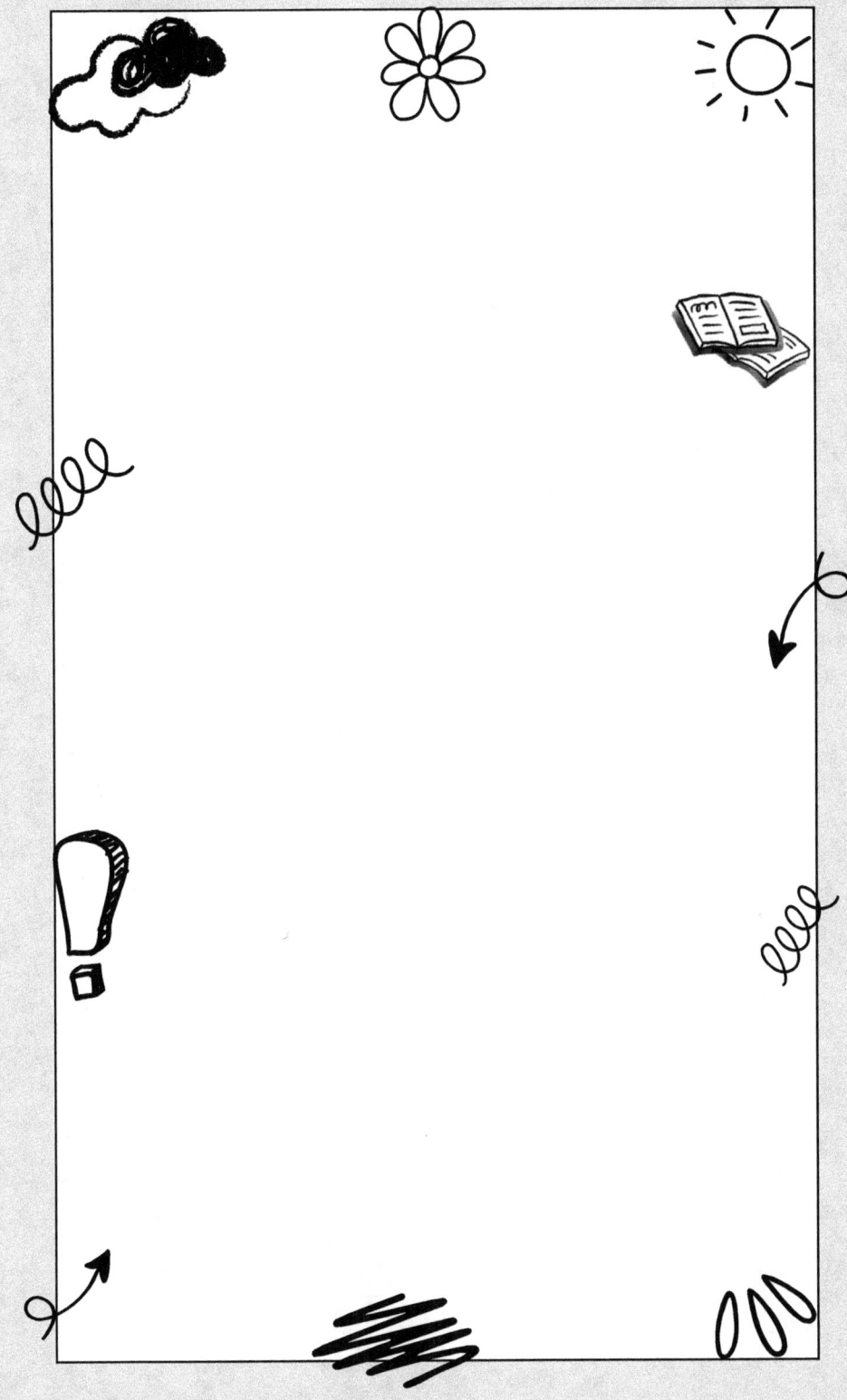

Chapter 6
NAMING MY NEEDS

Needs are not a burden; they are a guide to where you should be heading next.

Grounding routines and simple habits can gently support your body and mind. You don't need grand routines or rigid systems, what you need is something gentle, realistic and calming. This chapter offers small acts of care that you can return to when the days feel long or unsteady. Think of them as roots, that steady you while everything else moves around you. It's not about doing more, it's about finding rhythms that restore you.

We often think creativity is about making art, but really, it's about expression. Creativity can look like doodling, humming a tune, planting herbs, or writing down a thought. This is your invitation to create, not for anyone else, not to be perfect, but to reconnect with yourself.

Creativity opens a door back to yourself, it relieves stress, sparks joy and reminds you that you can still play and create beyond your role.

Small Self-Care Suggestion:

- Speak one need aloud, even if just to yourself.
- Practice saying 'no' to something today.

MY GENTLE GOAL FOR THIS CHAPTER

Find 5 minutes to be creative. You might use creative play, doodling, humming a song, or arranging something colourful on your table. Let it be light and fun, not a task.

One playful or creative act I will enjoy is …

How I'll know I honoured it:

I give myself permission to choose one simple thing that feels possible for me right now. It doesn't need to be big or perfect. Small is enough.

Moment for Reflection:

In what ways do I feel unseen?

What needs do I have that are unmet?

What do I need right now emotionally, physically, and spiritually?

GRATITUDE JOURNAL

The best part of the day was:
_____

3 good things that happened today:

- _____
- _____
- _____

People I'm grateful for:

- _____
- _____
- _____

3 things I'm grateful for today:

- _____
- _____
- _____

Tomorrow, I'm looking forward to:
_____
_____
_____

Moment for Reflection:

What daily rhythm in the morning, evening, or mealtimes could I build to gently support my sleep, thoughts, and mood?

SELF-CARE CHECKLIST

Self-care isn't just the act of ticking a box, it's a commitment to oneself. How did you look after yourself this week?

- [ ] Take a long bath
- [ ] Engage in a hobby
- [ ] Read for pleasure
- [ ] Listen to favorite music
- [ ] Go for a long walk
- [ ] Spend time with a friend
- [ ] Mindful meditation
- [ ] Watch a movie
- [ ] Journal thoughts
- [ ] Pamper yourself
- [ ] Try gentle yoga
- [ ] Take a short nap
- [ ] Cook a meal
- [ ] Go for a swim
- [ ] Visit a museum/gallery
- [ ] Practice gratitude
- [ ] Gardening
- [ ] Attend a workshop
- [ ] Paint or draw
- [ ] Explore a new place

Moment for Reflection:

Creativity doesn't need to be perfect, it only needs to be yours. May you permit yourself to play, explore, and express freely.

Moment for Reflection:

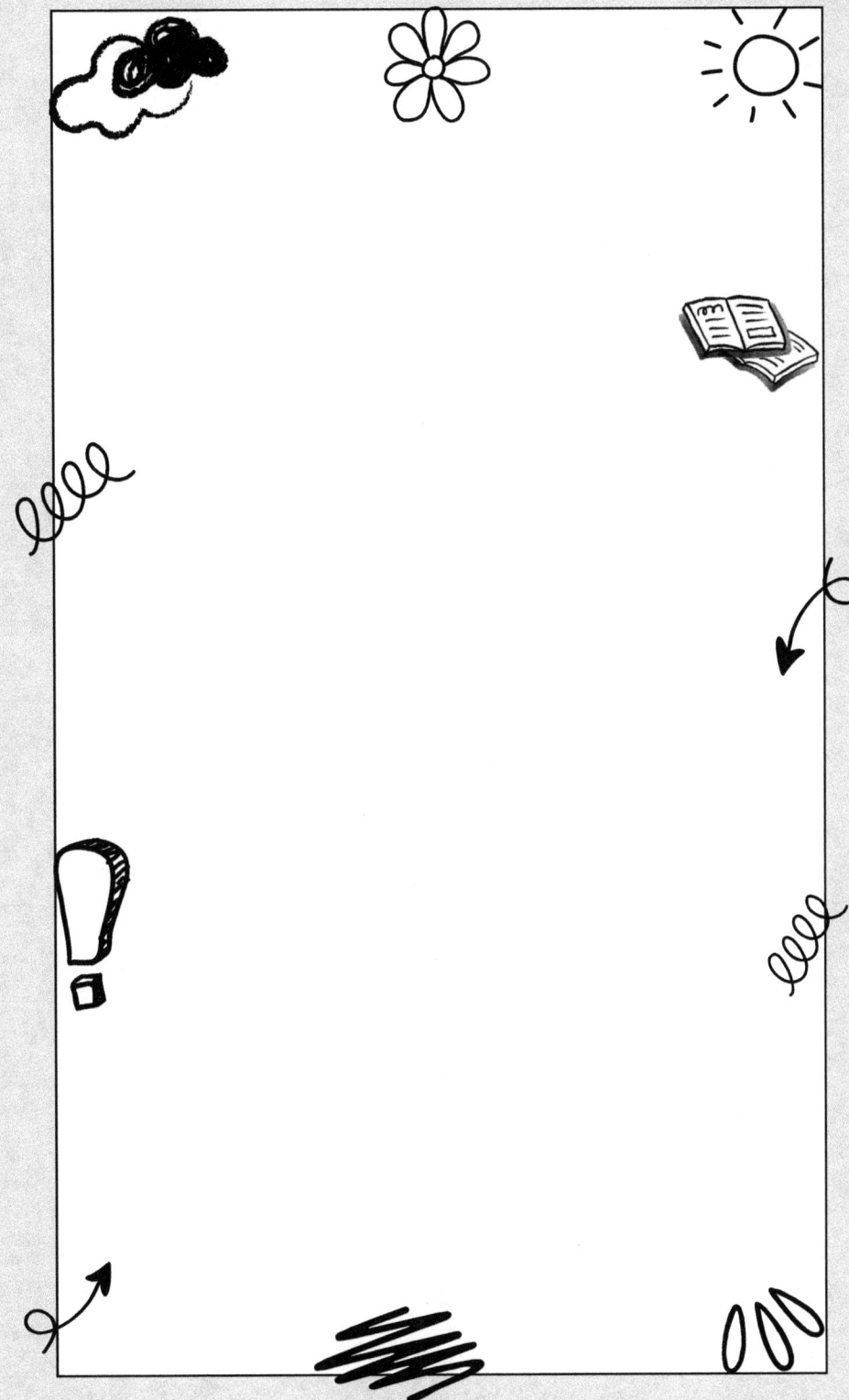

Chapter 7
GROWING THROUGH CHANGE

Some grief has no ceremony, only a quiet presence.

Even the strongest carers need care, and the most independent hearts need a hand to hold. This chapter is an invitation to reconnect with those you love, those you miss, and those you may have distanced from while surviving each day. It's also a space to honour the people who shaped you, including those who are no longer here.

Change is a constant companion in the caring journey. Some changes are expected, others are sudden, and many feel beyond our control. It is hoped you will see growth alongside change, not as a demand, but as a gentle noticing of how you are adapting, learning, and carrying resilience within you.

When you notice your own growth, even in hard times, you begin to see your resilience. Growth gives you confidence that you can keep moving forward. Noticing your own growth helps you see your own strength, something you may not have recognised, making future changes easier to carry.

> **Small Self-Care Suggestion:**
> Choose an object (blanket, scarf, a smooth stone) to hold as you sit quietly with your grief. You don't need to fix it, just be with it.

MY GENTLE GOAL FOR THIS CHAPTER

Growth is quiet and steady. Notice one small change in yourself this week, a thought, a feeling, or even a plant outside your window?

A small growth I will notice or nurture is …

How I'll know I honoured it:

I give myself permission to choose one simple thing that feels possible for me right now. It doesn't need to be big or perfect. Small is enough.

Moment for Reflection:

What am I grieving, even if others don't see it?

What unspoken grief am I holding in this season?

GRATITUDE JOURNAL

The best part of the day was:
_____

3 good things that happened today:

- _____
- _____
- _____

People I'm grateful for:

- _____
- _____
- _____

3 things I'm grateful for today:

- _____
- _____
- _____

Tomorrow, I'm looking forward to:
_____
_____
_____

Moment for Reflection:

Who in my life helps me feel mentally lighter, emotionally seen, or physically energised?

How might I connect with them this week, even in a small way?

SELF-CARE CHECKLIST

Self-care isn't just the act of ticking a box, it's a commitment to oneself. How did you look after yourself this week?

- [ ] Take a long bath
- [ ] Engage in a hobby
- [ ] Read for pleasure
- [ ] Listen to favorite music
- [ ] Go for a long walk
- [ ] Spend time with a friend
- [ ] Mindful meditation
- [ ] Watch a movie
- [ ] Journal thoughts
- [ ] Pamper yourself
- [ ] Try gentle yoga
- [ ] Take a short nap
- [ ] Cook a meal
- [ ] Go for a swim
- [ ] Visit a museum/gallery
- [ ] Practice gratitude
- [ ] Gardening
- [ ] Attend a workshop
- [ ] Paint or draw
- [ ] Explore a new place

Moment for Reflection:

Change is never easy, yet growth often blooms quietly in its shadow. May you notice the strength you carry within, even when you don't feel it.

Moment for Reflection:

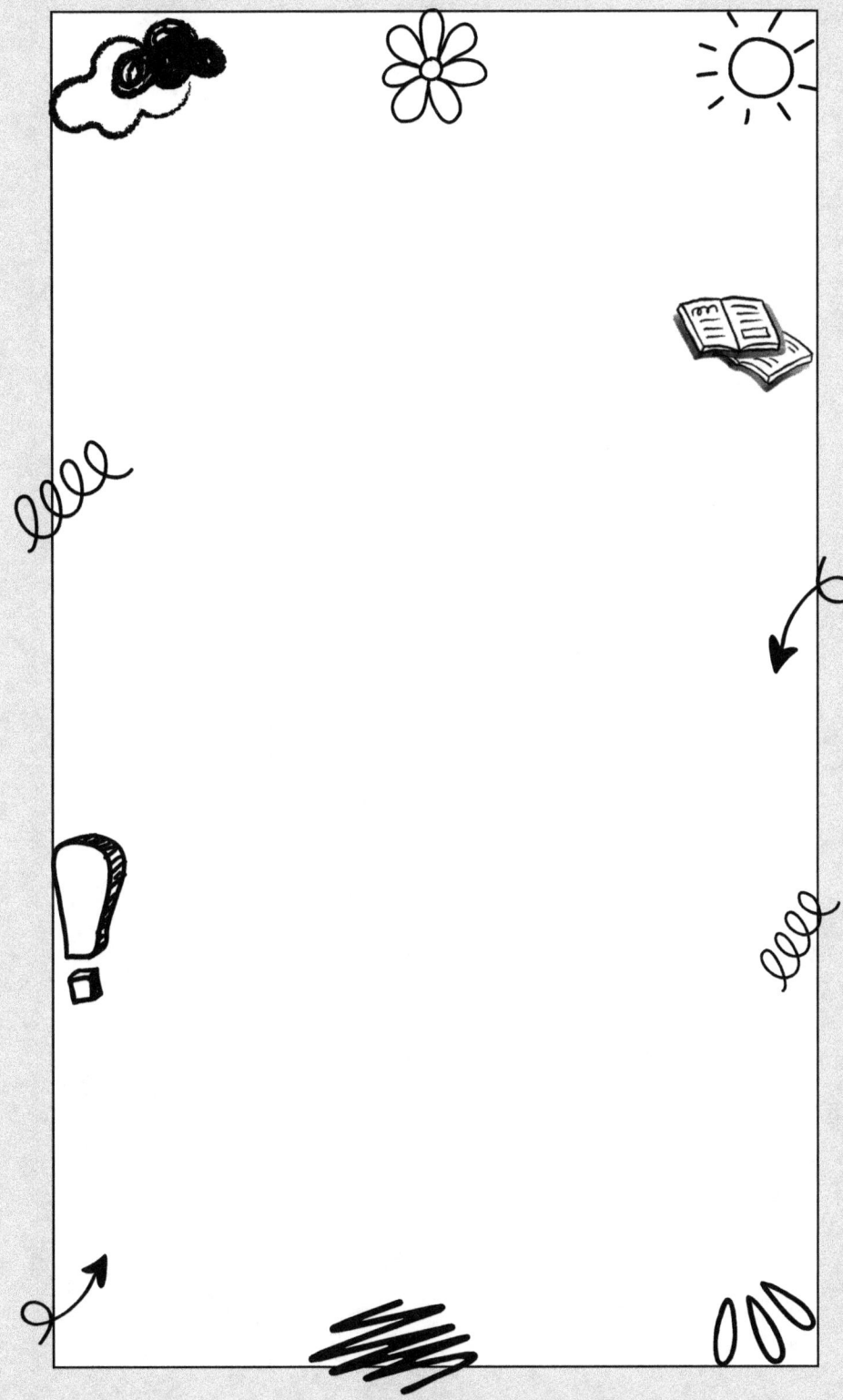

Chapter 8
PERMISSION TO FEEL IT ALL

You are allowed to feel everything. Even the messy, contradictory things.

There is healing in making, in scribbling, doodling, writing nonsense, making lists, colouring wildly, or drawing nothing in particular. You can be expressive without needing it to mean anything, to let your hand move before your mind catches up, to reconnect with play, with beauty, with creativity not as a luxury, but as a part of your healing and being human.

Connection sustains us, yet caring can sometimes feel isolating, as though the world has moved on without us. This chapter is about remembering the ties that matter, friendships, family bonds, shared laughter, and the small exchanges that remind you that you're not on your own.

Connection with others lessens loneliness and brings a sense of belonging. Sharing moments of care, laughter, or conversation can remind you that you're not walking this road alone. Staying connected reminds you that you're supported with those relationships bringing laughter, perspective, and comfort.

> **Small Self-Care Suggestion:**
>
> Set a timer for 10 minutes and free-write everything you're feeling, doing so with no edits and no judgment.

MY GENTLE GOAL FOR THIS CHAPTER

Connection doesn't have to be big, it might be one short text, one phone call, or a smile shared with someone nearby. Just one small thread of connection can be enough.

A moment of connection I will create is ...

How I'll know I honoured it:

I give myself permission to choose one simple thing that feels possible for me right now. It doesn't need to be big or perfect. Small is enough.

Moment for Reflection:

What am I noticing about myself today? (Remember there's no 'wrong' way to feel)

What am I feeling that I've been trying to suppress or hide?

GRATITUDE JOURNAL

The best part of the day was:
_____

3 good things that happened today:

- _____
- _____
- _____

People I'm grateful for:

- _____
- _____
- _____

3 things I'm grateful for today:

- _____
- _____
- _____

Tomorrow, I'm looking forward to:
_____
_____
_____

Moment for Reflection:

When I make something whether it's a drawing, writing something down, gardening or cooking, how does it shift my emotions, stress, or even the way my body feels?

SELF-CARE CHECKLIST

Self-care isn't just the act of ticking a box, it's a commitment to oneself. How did you look after yourself this week?

- [ ] Take a long bath
- [ ] Engage in a hobby
- [ ] Read for pleasure
- [ ] Listen to favorite music
- [ ] Go for a long walk
- [ ] Spend time with a friend
- [ ] Mindful meditation
- [ ] Watch a movie
- [ ] Journal thoughts
- [ ] Pamper yourself
- [ ] Try gentle yoga
- [ ] Take a short nap
- [ ] Cook a meal
- [ ] Go for a swim
- [ ] Visit a museum/gallery
- [ ] Practice gratitude
- [ ] Gardening
- [ ] Attend a workshop
- [ ] Paint or draw
- [ ] Explore a new place

Moment for Reflection:

You are not alone. May the bonds of love, memory, and friendship hold you in the moments you need them most.

Moment for Reflection:

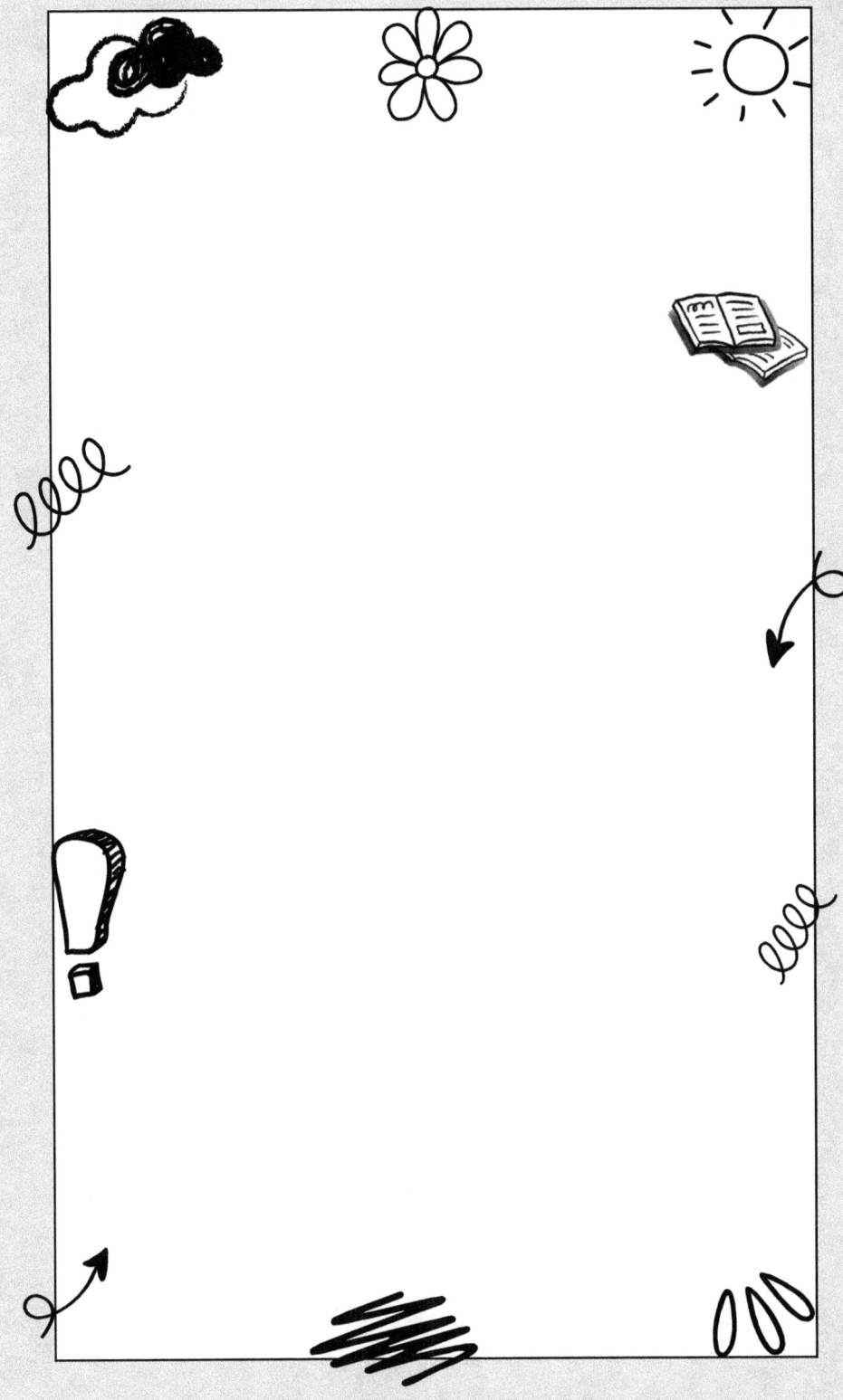

Chapter 9
WHAT REST LOOKS LIKE FOR ME

Rest is not earned, it is a necessity.

Some days, it's all too much and that's okay. These are the days that provide an opportunity to create some space and breathing room. They're not for reflection or action. They're for pausing. A time to close your eyes, place your hand on your heart without the need to solve anything, the granting of permission to 'just be'.

Letting go is not about forgetting. It's about releasing what no longer serves you, be it guilt, old expectations, or the need to do everything perfectly. This chapter encourages you to lighten your load gently, choosing what you can lay down while holding on to what still brings meaning.

Letting go of what weighs you down makes room for calm and freedom. Releasing guilt or expectations lightens your heart and restores peace, helping you feel lighter and freer.

Small Self-Care Suggestion:

Give yourself 15 minutes today with no agenda. Lie down, sip tea, look at the sky, just simply be in the moment.

MY GENTLE GOAL FOR THIS CHAPTER

Clear one small thing from your day, a thought, a worry, or even a single drawer? Release just one thing today.

One thing I will gently release is …

How I'll know I honoured it:

I give myself permission to choose one simple thing that feels possible for me right now. It doesn't need to be big or perfect. Small is enough.

Moment for Reflection:

What helps me feel rested, emotionally, mentally, and physically?

What does real rest feel like for me?

When did I last feel it?

GRATITUDE JOURNAL

The best part of the day was:
_____

3 good things that happened today:

- _____
- _____
- _____

People I'm grateful for:

- _____
- _____
- _____

3 things I'm grateful for today:

- _____
- _____
- _____

Tomorrow, I'm looking forward to:
_____
_____
_____

Moment for Reflection:

What do I notice in my body, mood, or mind after three slow breaths?

How might adding these pauses help my brain, body, or energy?

SELF-CARE CHECKLIST

Self-care isn't just the act of ticking a box, it's a commitment to oneself. How did you look after yourself this week?

- ☐ Take a long bath
- ☐ Engage in a hobby
- ☐ Read for pleasure
- ☐ Listen to favorite music
- ☐ Go for a long walk
- ☐ Spend time with a friend
- ☐ Mindful meditation
- ☐ Watch a movie
- ☐ Journal thoughts
- ☐ Pamper yourself
- ☐ Try gentle yoga
- ☐ Take a short nap
- ☐ Cook a meal
- ☐ Go for a swim
- ☐ Visit a museum/gallery
- ☐ Practice gratitude
- ☐ Gardening
- ☐ Attend a workshop
- ☐ Paint or draw
- ☐ Explore a new place

Moment for Reflection:

Letting go is an act of courage. May releasing what no longer serves you make room for gentleness, lightness, and new life.

Moment for Reflection:

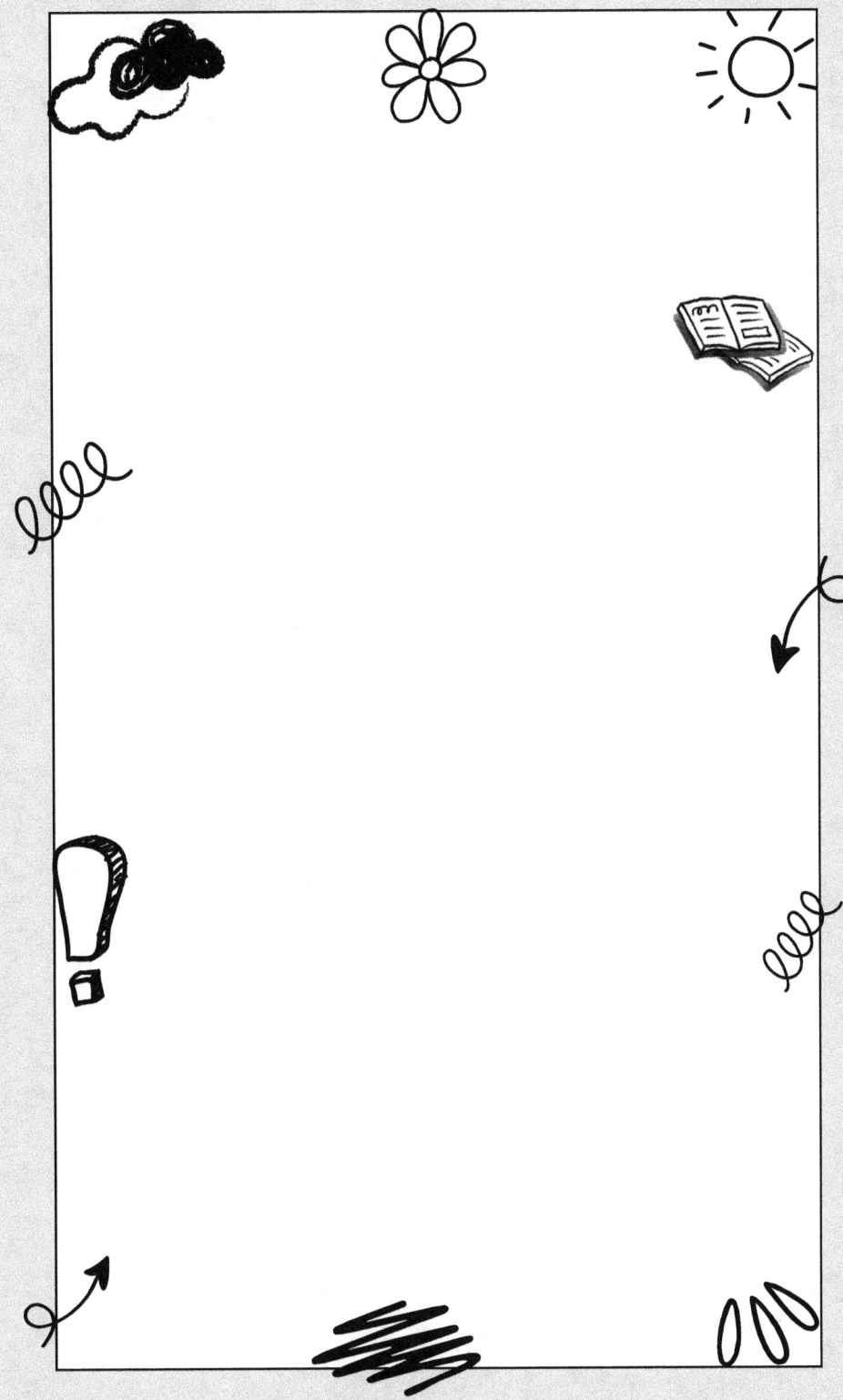

Chapter 10
TENDING TO MY FRAYED EDGES

You don't need to be everything to everyone. You only need to be gentle with yourself.

You are still becoming, even in this season, even after everything you have been managing. This chapter gently turns you toward the future, not with pressure or planning, but with possibility. You get to choose how you carry what you've learned and to reclaim parts of yourself. You get to keep becoming, not despite your caring journey, but shaped and strengthened by it.

Calm doesn't mean life is quiet or stress-free. It means you've found a small anchor, a breath, a ritual, or a practice that steadies you when things feel overwhelming. This anchor can help you explore the little things that bring calm back to your centre.

Calm practices soothe your nervous system and steady your mind. They can help you feel more present, more balanced, and better able to care without burning out. Practising calm reduces overwhelm. When your nervous system relaxes, your thoughts clear, and you regain steadiness for yourself and those you care for.

> **Small Self-Care Suggestion:**
>
> Do something nurturing for your senses: hand cream, warm socks, soft music, a favourite scent.

MY GENTLE GOAL FOR THIS CHAPTER

Try something just once this week like sitting in the garden listening to birds, holding a warm mug, or closing your eyes in stillness.

One calming practice I will try is ...

How I'll know I honoured it:

I give myself permission to choose one simple thing that feels possible for me right now. It doesn't need to be big or perfect. Small is enough.

Moment for Reflection:

What might help me soften and mend?

Where do I feel like I'm fraying?

What needs tending?

GRATITUDE JOURNAL

The best part of the day was:
_____

3 good things that happened today:

- _____
- _____
- _____

People I'm grateful for:

- _____
- _____
- _____

3 things I'm grateful for today:

- _____
- _____
- _____

Tomorrow, I'm looking forward to:
_____
_____
_____

Moment for Reflection:

As I imagine my future self, what routines or relationships do I hope will support my mind, body, and heart?

What helps me feel calm for even one minute?

SELF-CARE CHECKLIST

Self-care isn't just the act of ticking a box, it's a commitment to oneself. How did you look after yourself this week?

- [ ] Take a long bath
- [ ] Read for pleasure
- [ ] Go for a long walk
- [ ] Mindful meditation
- [ ] Journal thoughts
- [ ] Try gentle yoga
- [ ] Cook a meal
- [ ] Visit a museum/gallery
- [ ] Gardening
- [ ] Paint or draw
- [ ] Engage in a hobby
- [ ] Listen to favorite music
- [ ] Spend time with a friend
- [ ] Watch a movie
- [ ] Pamper yourself
- [ ] Take a short nap
- [ ] Go for a swim
- [ ] Practice gratitude
- [ ] Attend a workshop
- [ ] Explore a new place

Moment for Reflection:

Calm doesn't erase the storm, but it gives you an anchor. May you carry this anchor into the days ahead, steady and sure.

Moment for Reflection:

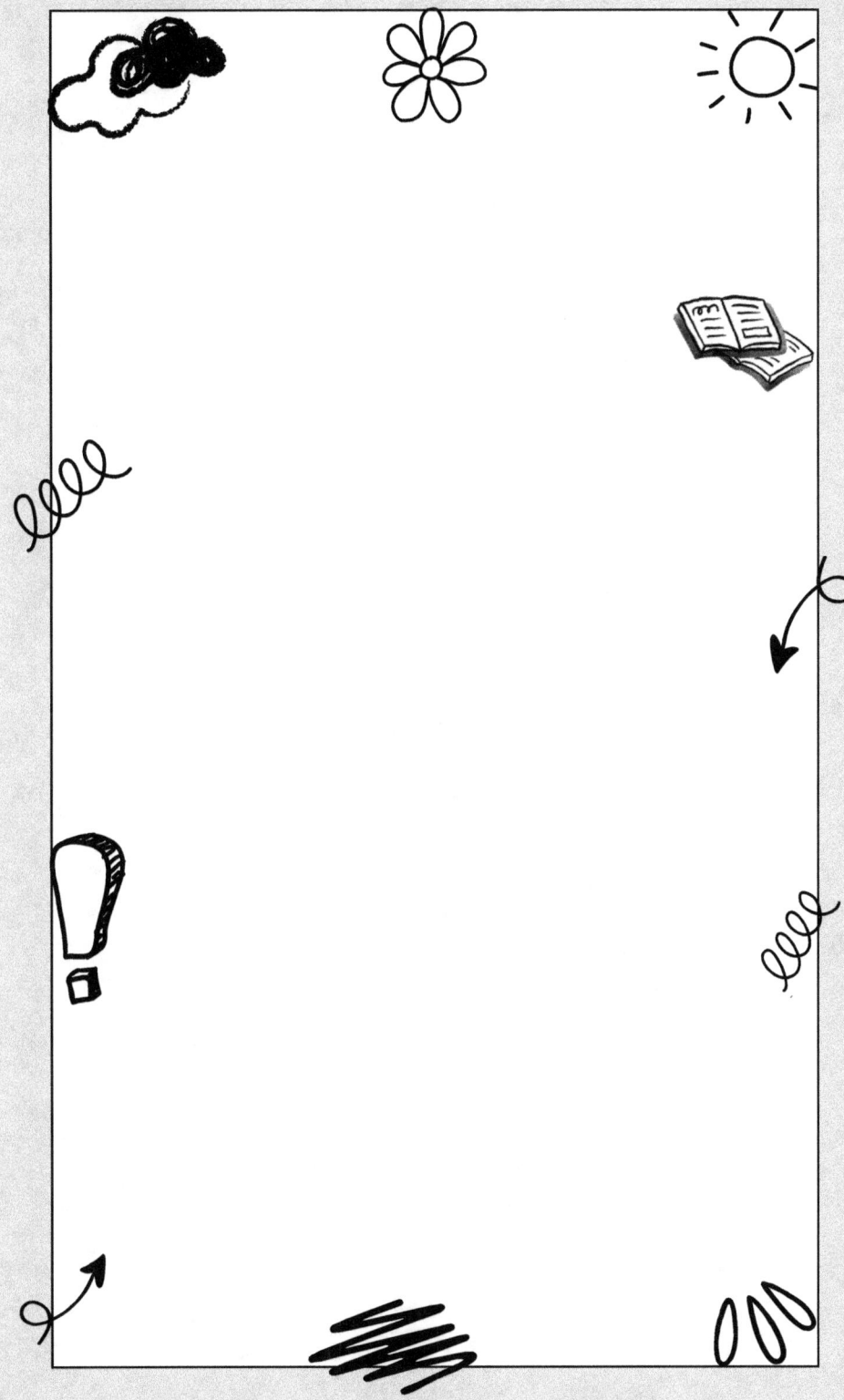

Chapter 11
LITTLE JOYS, BIG IMPACT

Joy doesn't need to be loud, it can live quietly in the corners of your day.

When everything feels heavy, it's easy to miss the soft, quiet joys around us - a bird outside the window, a patch of sun on the floor, a sentence that makes you feel understood. This chapter is a reminder to look for beauty not in big fixes, but in the small things that so often get overlooked. You don't have to feel grateful all the time, but sometimes, noticing one small thing that sparks joy can anchor you back to yourself.

Caring takes energy, sometimes more than feels possible, renewal is about noticing where your energy is spent and gently choosing ways to restore it. This is a time to think about tiny sparks, moments of laughter, rest, or nourishment that help refill your inner cup.

Replenishing and tending to your energy can help prevent exhaustion, it works towards bringing back your spark, making it possible to keep giving without losing yourself. When you restore your energy, you not only prevent burnout, but also protect your overall health.

Small Self-Care Suggestion:

Create a 'joy jar' and add a slip of paper each time something makes you smile.

MY GENTLE GOAL FOR THIS CHAPTER

Energy doesn't come from doing more, it comes from small intentional choices. Your goal could be to drink an extra glass of water, or take a short rest without guilt. Just one renewing act.

A choice that renews my energy will be …

How I'll know I honoured it:

I give myself permission to choose one simple thing that feels possible for me right now. It doesn't need to be big or perfect. Small is enough.

Moment for Reflection:

What small things bring light into my day?

What small thing brought me a moment of lightness this week?

GRATITUDE JOURNAL

The best part of the day was:
_____

3 good things that happened today:

- _____
- _____
- _____

People I'm grateful for:

- _____
- _____
- _____

3 things I'm grateful for today:

- _____
- _____
- _____

Tomorrow, I'm looking forward to:
_____
_____
_____

Moment for Reflection:

What small moment today brought me joy, the sunlight, a flower, a sip of tea?

How did it affect my mood or body?

SELF-CARE CHECKLIST

Self-care isn't just the act of ticking a box, it's a commitment to oneself. How did you look after yourself this week?

- [ ] Take a long bath
- [ ] Engage in a hobby
- [ ] Read for pleasure
- [ ] Listen to favorite music
- [ ] Go for a long walk
- [ ] Spend time with a friend
- [ ] Mindful meditation
- [ ] Watch a movie
- [ ] Journal thoughts
- [ ] Pamper yourself
- [ ] Try gentle yoga
- [ ] Take a short nap
- [ ] Cook a meal
- [ ] Go for a swim
- [ ] Visit a museum/gallery
- [ ] Practice gratitude
- [ ] Gardening
- [ ] Attend a workshop
- [ ] Paint or draw
- [ ] Explore a new place

Moment for Reflection:

Energy ebbs and flows. May you welcome renewal in small sparks, moments that light your spirit and refill your heart.

Moment for Reflection:

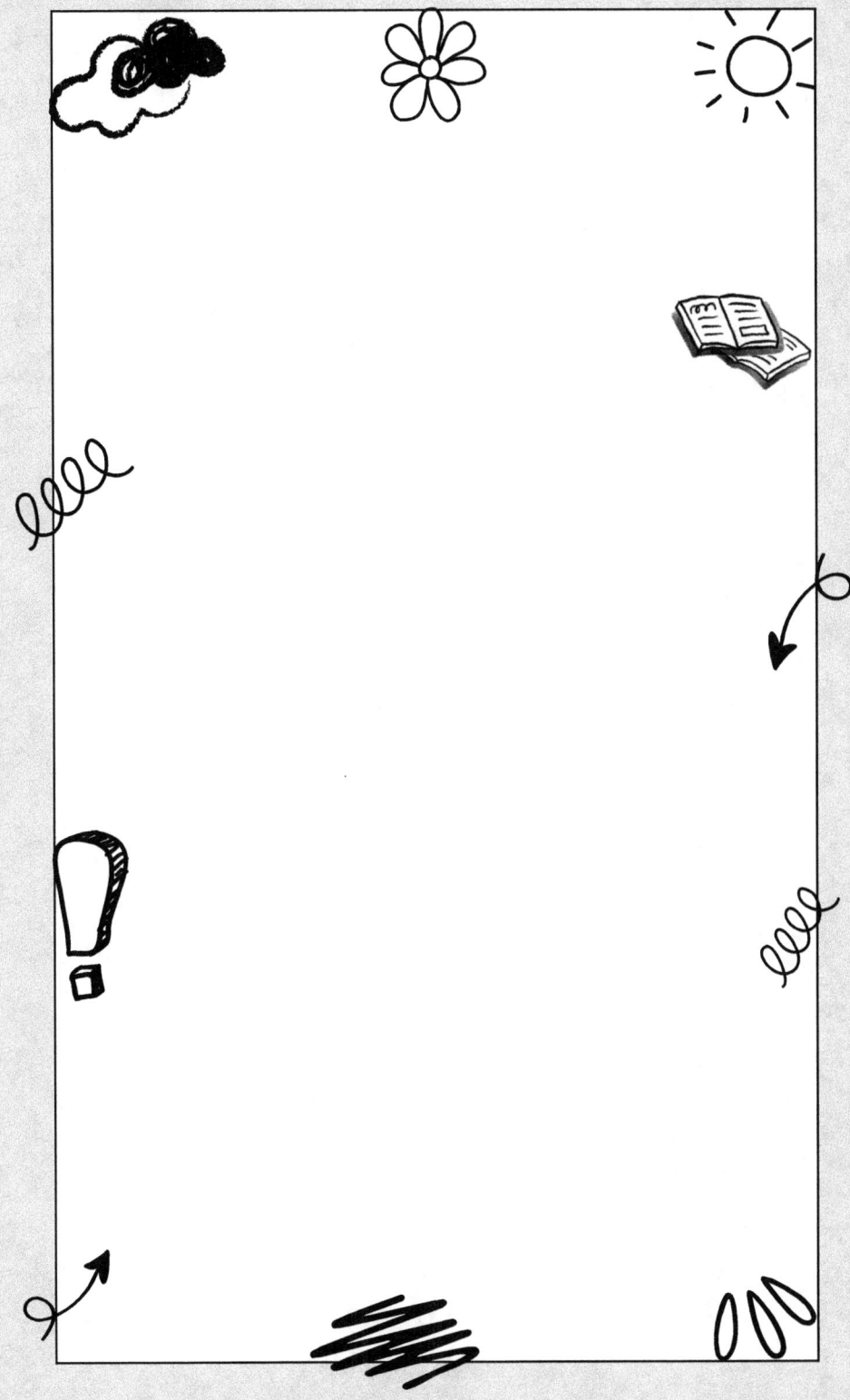

Chapter 12
BOUNDARIES ARE KINDNESS

A boundary is not a wall, it is a doorway into your own wellbeing.

Caring often carries a quiet grief; grief for the person you once knew, grief for the life you have paused, the grief that lives right alongside love. You don't have to choose between hope and heartache; you're allowed to feel it all. But to do so means first setting boundaries to allow time for the things that really matter. The simple act of saying 'no' to others can be saying 'yes' to time spent on yourself.

Nature has a way of reminding us of cycles, resilience, and beauty. A single flower, a patch of sunlight, or the sound of rain can soothe us when words cannot. This chapter invites you to let nature hold you, even if only for a few minutes each day.

Small moments with nature lower stress and lift mood. Nature helps you feel grounded, reminding you of cycles of rest, growth, and renewal. Spending time in nature lowers stress, boosts mood, and calms the body. Small doses of sunlight, fresh air, or greenery can lift your spirit.

> **Small Self-Care Suggestion:**
> Practice saying and setting a kind but firm boundary out loud. Or write a list of things you no longer have to say 'yes' to.

MY GENTLE GOAL FOR THIS CHAPTER

Notice something natural around you today, the sky, a flower, a tree. You don't have to travel far, let nature come to you in small moments.

A moment with nature I will welcome is ...

How I'll know I honoured it:

I give myself permission to choose one simple thing that feels possible for me right now. It doesn't need to be big or perfect. Small is enough.

Moment for Reflection:

What boundary do I need to hold for myself this week?

Where in my life do I need firmer boundaries to protect my energy?

GRATITUDE JOURNAL

The best part of the day was:
_____

3 good things that happened today:

- _____
- _____
- _____

People I'm grateful for:

- _____
- _____
- _____

3 things I'm grateful for today:

- _____
- _____
- _____

Tomorrow, I'm looking forward to:
_____
_____
_____

Moment for Reflection:

What rituals and/or connections bring me comfort in grief, and how do they also care for my health?

SELF-CARE CHECKLIST

Self-care isn't just the act of ticking a box, it's a commitment to oneself. How did you look after yourself this week?

- ☐ Take a long bath
- ☐ Engage in a hobby
- ☐ Read for pleasure
- ☐ Listen to favorite music
- ☐ Go for a long walk
- ☐ Spend time with a friend
- ☐ Mindful meditation
- ☐ Watch a movie
- ☐ Journal thoughts
- ☐ Pamper yourself
- ☐ Try gentle yoga
- ☐ Take a short nap
- ☐ Cook a meal
- ☐ Go for a swim
- ☐ Visit a museum/gallery
- ☐ Practice gratitude
- ☐ Gardening
- ☐ Attend a workshop
- ☐ Paint or draw
- ☐ Explore a new place

Moment for Reflection:

Nature holds wisdom in its rhythms. May you let the earth remind you that rest, growth, and renewal are all part of the same cycle.

Moment for Reflection:

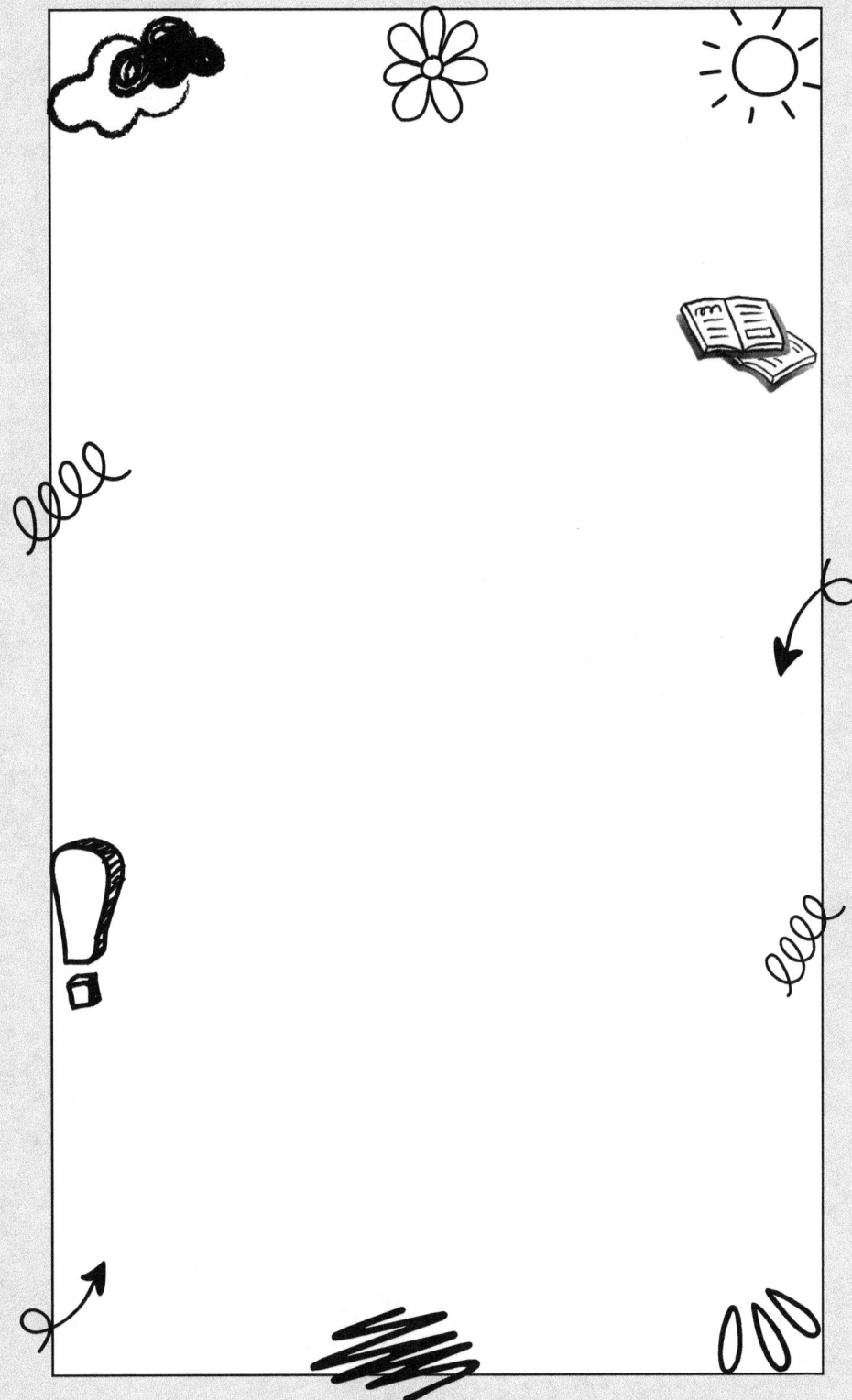

Chapter 13
TINY SPARKS OF HOPE

The smallest ray of light can change the shape of the dark.

Before the schedules, medication charts, and waiting rooms, there was you. A person who made plans for the weekend, who had a favourite band, special friendships, and a future dream. This chapter welcomes the dreamer in you back, not as a return to the past, but as a remembering of who you still are and reclaim the parts of you that have been set aside.

Rest is not a weakness. It's a necessity, and yet carers often feel guilty for slowing down. You're encouraged to see rest as a gift, a form of strength, and a way to restore yourself. Rest doesn't always mean sleep; sometimes it just means stillness.

Rest restores your body, clears your mind, and renews your spirit. It gives you strength to carry on without losing or sacrificing your own health. It allows you to care from a place of strength rather than exhaustion. Rest gives you permission to slow down and say that you've done enough for today.

Small Self-Care Suggestion:

Make a playlist of songs that lift your spirit, even if just a little.

MY GENTLE GOAL FOR THIS CHAPTER

Rest can be simple, your goal might be one early night, a nap, or even sitting with your feet up for five minutes. That alone can be enough.

One way I will rest this week is ...

How I'll know I honoured it:

I give myself permission to choose one simple thing that feels possible for me right now. It doesn't need to be big or perfect. Small is enough.

Moment for Reflection:

What activities or foods from my past have helped me feel strong, creative, or alive?

Could revisiting them support my health now?

GRATITUDE JOURNAL

The best part of the day was:
_____

3 good things that happened today:

- _____
- _____
- _____

People I'm grateful for:

- _____
- _____
- _____

3 things I'm grateful for today:

- _____
- _____
- _____

Tomorrow, I'm looking forward to:
_____
_____
_____

Moment for Reflection:

What's giving me even the faintest glimmer of hope and joy right now?

SELF-CARE CHECKLIST

Self-care isn't just the act of ticking a box, it's a commitment to oneself. How did you look after yourself this week?

- ☐ Take a long bath
- ☐ Read for pleasure
- ☐ Go for a long walk
- ☐ Mindful meditation
- ☐ Journal thoughts
- ☐ Try gentle yoga
- ☐ Cook a meal
- ☐ Visit a museum/gallery
- ☐ Gardening
- ☐ Paint or draw

- ☐ Engage in a hobby
- ☐ Listen to favorite music
- ☐ Spend time with a friend
- ☐ Watch a movie
- ☐ Pamper yourself
- ☐ Take a short nap
- ☐ Go for a swim
- ☐ Practice gratitude
- ☐ Attend a workshop
- ☐ Explore a new place

Moment for Reflection:

Rest is not indulgence, it is healing. May you allow yourself to be restored in ways both simple and profound.

Moment for Reflection:

Chapter 14
MOMENTS I WANT TO KEEP

There is beauty, even here, especially here.

Memories are fragile, but they also carry gifts. While dementia changes memory for a person, it doesn't take everything, memories can be places of comfort and grounding. This chapter invites you to reflect on the memories you hold dear, and to treasure them as part of who you are.

Memories reconnect you with joy, meaning, and identity. Remembering what matters most helps you feel whole. It reminds you of who you are, beyond caring, and can strengthen your resilience.

Small Self-Care Suggestion:

Write down a memory that brings you joy in as much detail as you can. Let it live on the page and in your heart.

MY GENTLE GOAL FOR THIS CHAPTER

Choose one memory to treasure this week, your goal might be to write it down, tell it to someone, or simply sit with it in your heart.

One memory I will treasure this week is …

How I'll know I honoured it:

I give myself permission to choose one simple thing that feels possible for me right now. It doesn't need to be big or perfect. Small is enough.

Moment for Reflection:

What moment felt like love or truth this week?

GRATITUDE JOURNAL

The best part of the day was:
_____

3 good things that happened today:

- _____
- _____
- _____

People I'm grateful for:

- _____
- _____
- _____

3 things I'm grateful for today:

- _____
- _____
- _____

Tomorrow, I'm looking forward to:
_____
_____
_____

Moment for Reflection:

What moment this week felt meaningful, even if no one else saw it?

SELF-CARE CHECKLIST

Self-care isn't just the act of ticking a box, it's a commitment to oneself. How did you look after yourself this week?

- [ ] Take a long bath
- [ ] Engage in a hobby
- [ ] Read for pleasure
- [ ] Listen to favorite music
- [ ] Go for a long walk
- [ ] Spend time with a friend
- [ ] Mindful meditation
- [ ] Watch a movie
- [ ] Journal thoughts
- [ ] Pamper yourself
- [ ] Try gentle yoga
- [ ] Take a short nap
- [ ] Cook a meal
- [ ] Go for a swim
- [ ] Visit a museum/gallery
- [ ] Practice gratitude
- [ ] Gardening
- [ ] Attend a workshop
- [ ] Paint or draw
- [ ] Explore a new place

Moment for Reflection:

Memories can be both tender and strong. May the ones you hold close bring comfort, warmth, and a reminder of who you are.

Moment for Reflection:

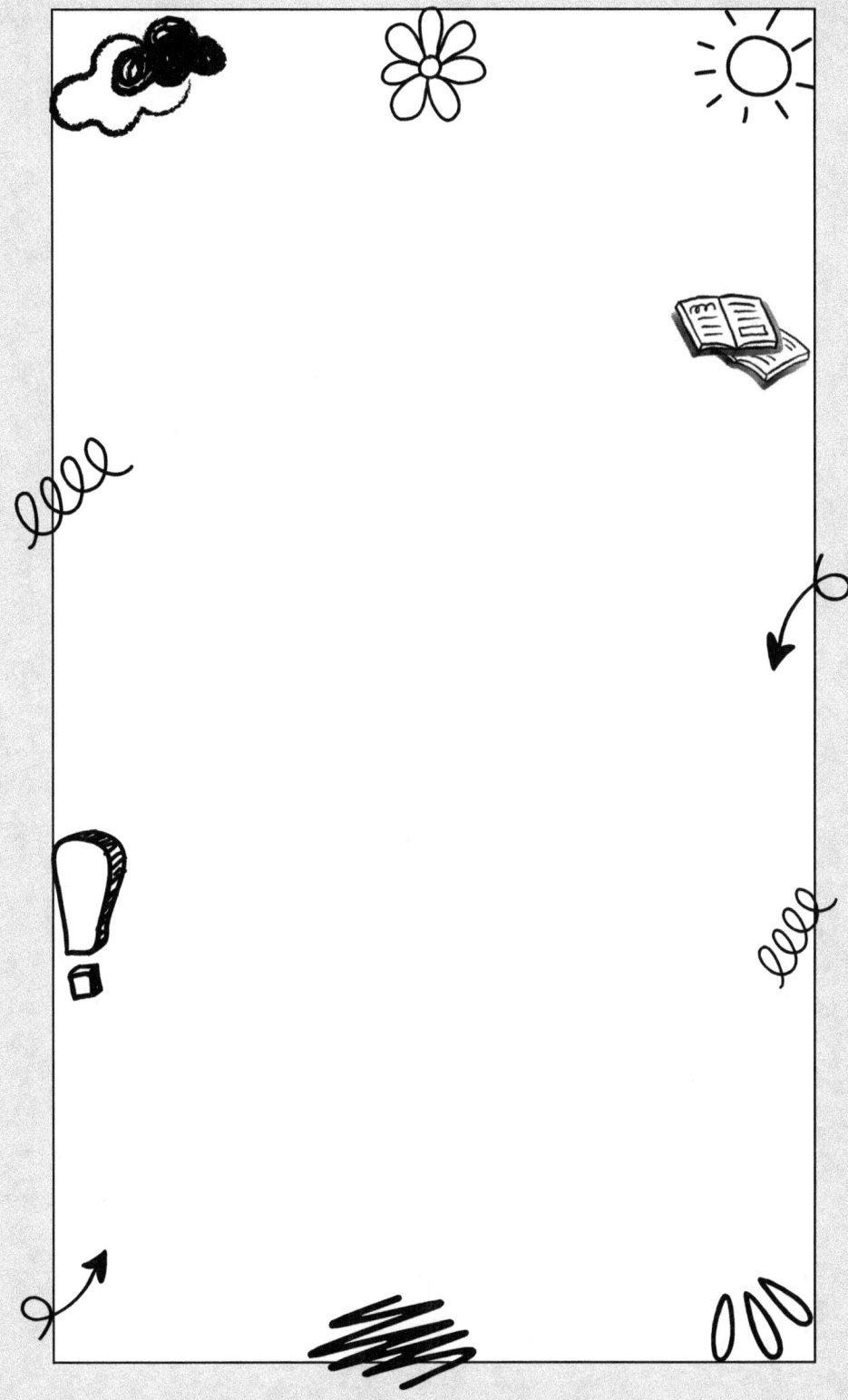

Chapter 15
WHAT I STILL DREAM ABOUT

You don't have to let go of your dreams to care for others.
You just need to keep them close.

You may feel alone in this journey, but you're not. There are others walking a similar path, quietly, bravely, and imperfectly too. This journal was created with you in mind, for your story. You belong here, not for what you do, but for who you are.

Honouring yourself outside your role helps to rebuild balance. Remember that you are more than the care you give. You are a person, with dreams, loves, talents, and a life that matters outside of your role. This chapter is a gentle reminder to reconnect with yourself, to rediscover parts of your identity that may feel hidden beneath caring, to give yourself permission to keep growing and living as your own person.

Small Self-Care Suggestion:

Write down a dream you still carry for yourself big or small:
- A trip you hope to take, a class you'd like to try, a garden you'd love to grow. What one tiny step could you take to keep that dream alive?
- Look up a recipe from the country you want visit, or buy a packet of seeds for the flowers you imagine?

MY GENTLE GOAL FOR THIS CHAPTER

Do one thing that feels like 'you'. Listening to your favourite music, wearing your favourite colour, or reading one page of a book you've always wanted to read.

One thing I will do just for me is ...

How I'll know I honoured it:

I give myself permission to choose one simple thing that feels possible for me right now. It doesn't need to be big or perfect. Small is enough.

Moment for Reflection:

Even now, I carry dreams. What are they?

What do I still long for?

What dreams feel alive inside me?

GRATITUDE JOURNAL

The best part of the day was:
_____

3 good things that happened today:

- _____
- _____
- _____

People I'm grateful for:

- _____
- _____
- _____

3 things I'm grateful for today:

- _____
- _____
- _____

Tomorrow, I'm looking forward to:
_____
_____
_____

Moment for Reflection:

Where do I feel most connected, at a table, in a garden, on a walk, with others?

How does that connection support my health?

SELF-CARE CHECKLIST

Self-care isn't just the act of ticking a box, it's a commitment to oneself. How did you look after yourself this week?

- ☐ Take a long bath
- ☐ Engage in a hobby
- ☐ Read for pleasure
- ☐ Listen to favorite music
- ☐ Go for a long walk
- ☐ Spend time with a friend
- ☐ Mindful meditation
- ☐ Watch a movie
- ☐ Journal thoughts
- ☐ Pamper yourself
- ☐ Try gentle yoga
- ☐ Take a short nap
- ☐ Cook a meal
- ☐ Go for a swim
- ☐ Visit a museum/gallery
- ☐ Practice gratitude
- ☐ Gardening
- ☐ Attend a workshop
- ☐ Paint or draw
- ☐ Explore a new place

Moment for Reflection:

You are more than your role. May you rediscover the parts of yourself that shine quietly beneath, waiting to be seen again.

Moment for Reflection:

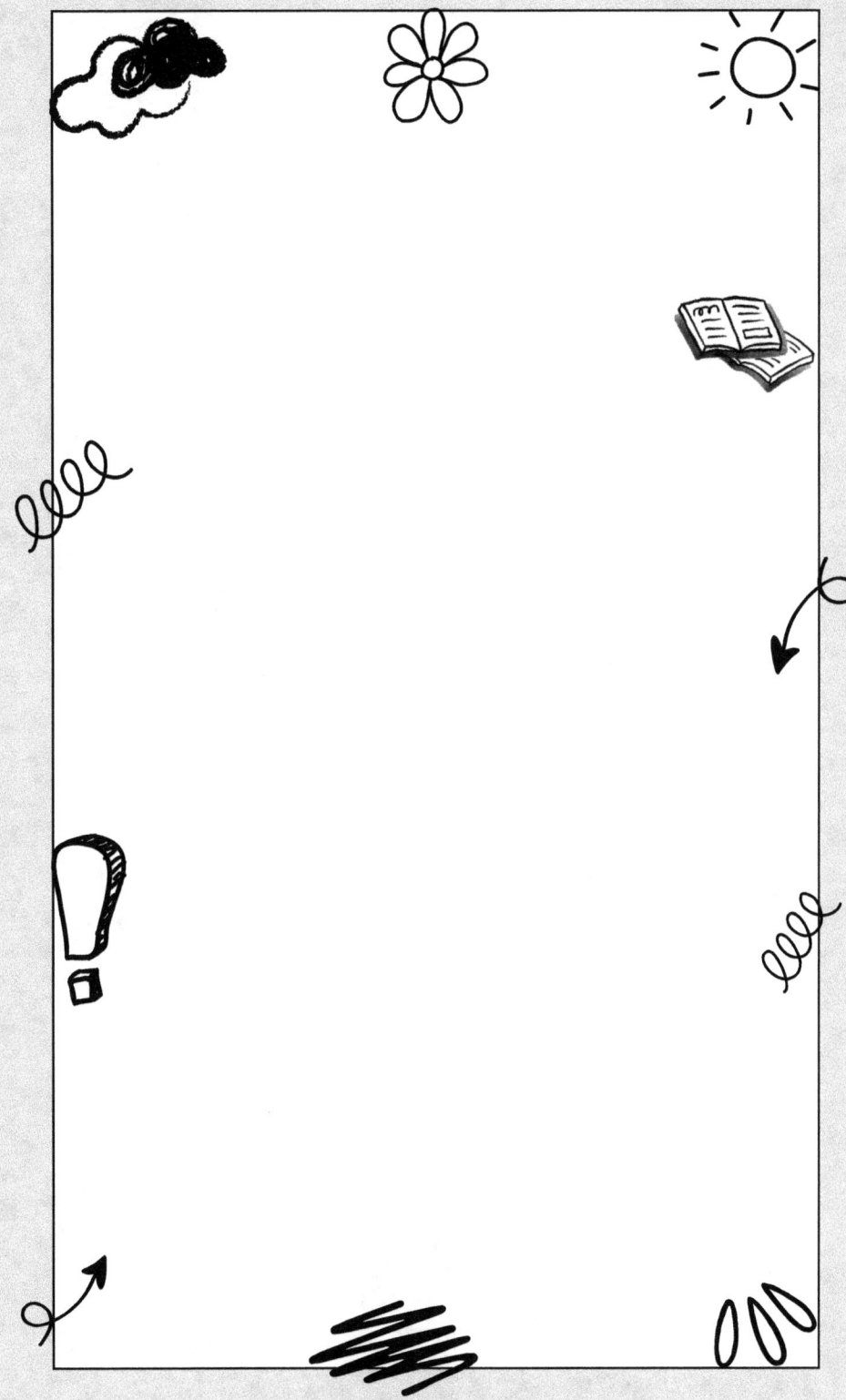

Chapter 16
LIFE BEYOND THE ROLE

When this season changes, your next chapter will begin.

The future can feel uncertain, but it also holds possibility. Looking ahead doesn't mean having everything figured out. It means continuing to hope, imagining what life could be, and honouring that there is still more of you to come. This chapter is about moving forward with softness and strength knowing that with every page of your story, every pause, every tear and breath, something inside you will continue to shift and grow.

You're growing not because you're trying harder, but because you're allowing yourself to be whole. By holding a space for the new you that is quietly forming, one shaped by love, loss, courage, and deep care, you hold hope for a future that may make today feel just a little bit lighter. Looking ahead gives you purpose, courage, and a sense of possibility beyond the present moment.

Holding hope for the future creates resilience in the present. Looking ahead can help you feel less stuck in today and opens space for possibility. There's no rush to arrive, 'becoming' always takes time.

> **Small Self-Care Suggestion:**
>
> Create a 'future me' vision board or journal page on what you want more of in your next chapter?

MY GENTLE GOAL FOR THIS CHAPTER

Looking ahead doesn't mean planning everything or giving up on today. Your goal could be to write one hope, one word, or one small wish for your future self, just one is enough.

One hope or wish I will carry forward is ...

How I'll know I honoured it:

I give myself permission to choose one simple thing that feels possible for me right now. It doesn't need to be big or perfect. Small is enough.

Moment for Reflection:

When this role shifts, who do I want to be?

What parts of me do I want to carry forward?

GRATITUDE JOURNAL

The best part of the day was:

_____

3 good things that happened today:

- _____
- _____
- _____

People I'm grateful for:

- _____
- _____
- _____

3 things I'm grateful for today:

- _____
- _____
- _____

Tomorrow, I'm looking forward to:

_____

_____

_____

Moment for Reflection:

How does looking at the future help me today?

What have I learned about myself that I will take forward into my next chapter?

What will I leave behind?

SELF-CARE CHECKLIST

Self-care isn't just the act of ticking a box, it's a commitment to oneself. How did you look after yourself this week?

- ☐ Take a long bath
- ☐ Read for pleasure
- ☐ Go for a long walk
- ☐ Mindful meditation
- ☐ Journal thoughts
- ☐ Try gentle yoga
- ☐ Cook a meal
- ☐ Visit a museum/gallery
- ☐ Gardening
- ☐ Paint or draw
- ☐ Engage in a hobby
- ☐ Listen to favorite music
- ☐ Spend time with a friend
- ☐ Watch a movie
- ☐ Pamper yourself
- ☐ Take a short nap
- ☐ Go for a swim
- ☐ Practice gratitude
- ☐ Attend a workshop
- ☐ Explore a new place

Moment for Reflection:

The future is unwritten, and hope belongs to me. May I step forward with gentleness, knowing that more of my story is still unfolding.

Moment for Reflection:

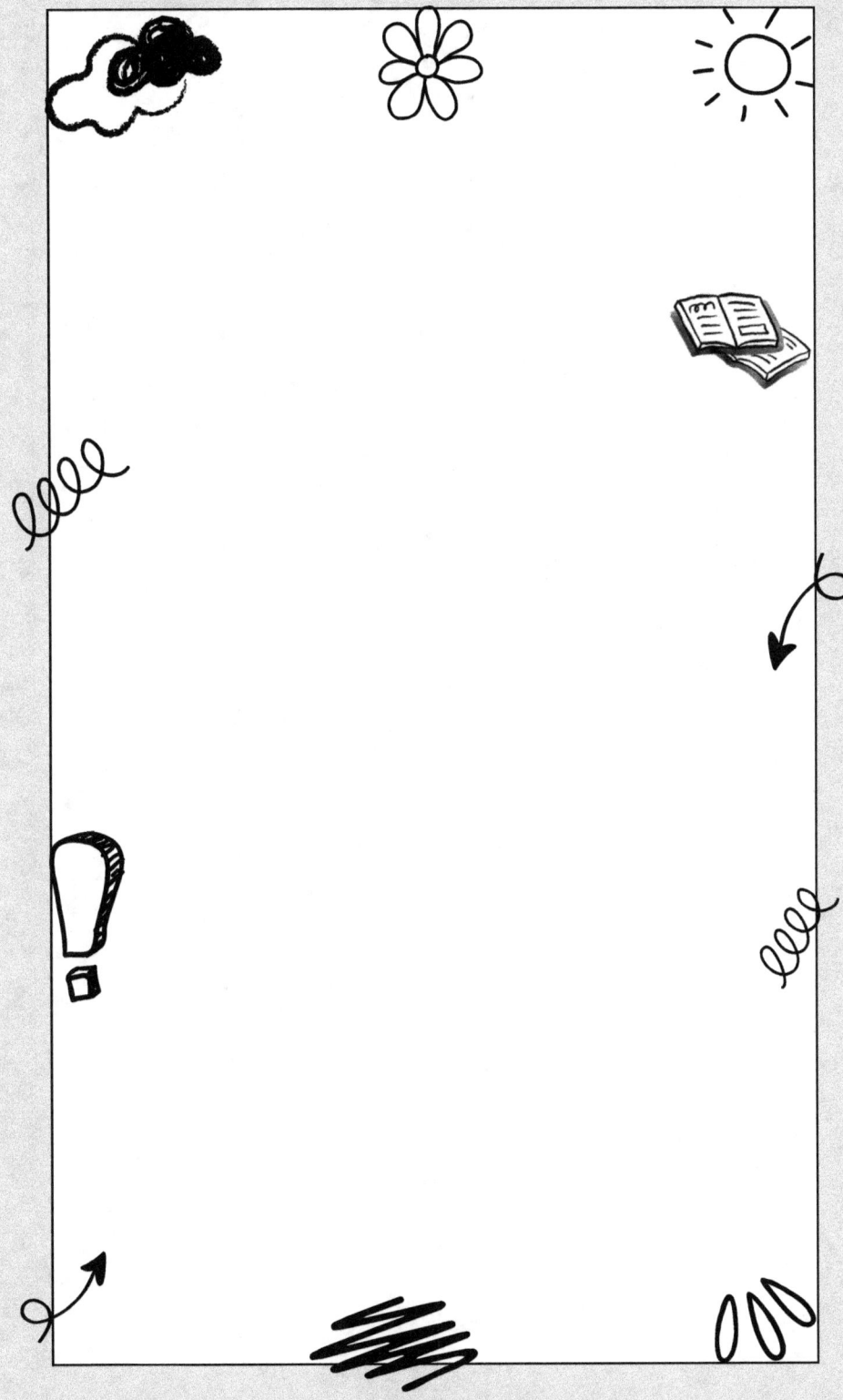

Dear Future Me,

I hope this letter finds you resting in the soft light of a slower morning, breathing more deeply than you have in a while. Right now, you are carrying so much. You're doing your best to be strong, to be gentle, to hold it all together for someone who may not always see how much of yourself you give. But I want you to know I see you. I remember every quiet act of love, every late night, every moment you pushed through your own exhaustion to ease someone else's pain.

But I also know this: You were always more than the care you gave, and you still are. There will come a time when the role of 'carer' will no longer consume your days. And while that may feel impossible now, or too painful to imagine, I promise, the space that opens will not be empty. It will be tender ground for rediscovery. It will be where you meet yourself again. The self who laughed freely, the self who had longings and ideas and weekend plans, the self who danced in the kitchen or wrote poems in the margins.

You are not just surviving this; you are growing through it. The compassion, courage, and wisdom you're building now will shape the life that waits you on the other side. You may carry grief, you may carry love that no longer has a place to land, but you will also carry your own name again and that name is worth remembering.

With love and fierce hope, the you who never disappeared, the one waiting to be found again.

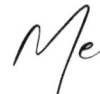

www.ingramcontent.com/pod-product-compliance
Lightning Source LLC
Chambersburg PA
CBHW072005290426
44109CB00018B/2134